CLOUDY URINE

FEW STEPS THAT HELPED ME TREAT
CLOUDY URINE

DR. J. SIMON

Contents

INTRODUCTION

Urine that looks murky or hazy instead of clear is referred to as cloudy pee. It is possible that there are multiple reasons for the cloudiness, and it occasionally suggests a medical condition. A persistent cloudiness or accompanying symptoms may indicate that additional research is necessary, even though occasional cloudy pee is probably nothing to worry about.

The following are typical reasons for murky urine:

Dehydration: Cloudy pee can result from concentrated urine.

Urinary Tract Infection (UTI): Painful, frequent, and uncomfortable urinating are possible signs of bacterial infections in the urinary tract, which can also result in murky urine.

Cloudy urine may be caused by kidney stones, which are characterized by the presence of crystals or particles in the urine.

Sexually transmitted infections, or STIs, can result in cloudy urine and are frequently accompanied by additional symptoms. Examples of these infections include gonorrhea and chlamydia.

Proteinuria: An abundance of protein in the urine may be linked to kidney issues and present as cloudiness.

Urinary cloudiness, urgency, and discomfort can all be symptoms of bladder infections.

Some Drugs: Urine color and clarity may vary as a result of taking certain drugs or supplements.

Changes in the appearance of urine can occur during pregnancy due to hormonal changes.

It is noteworthy to mention that certain meals, like asparagus, can also momentarily alter the color and clarity of urine.

A trip to the doctor is necessary if there are persistent cloudiness or other symptoms, even though occasional cloudiness in the urine may be normal. The underlying cause may be found by doing diagnostic testing, such as urinalysis. It's essential to consult a doctor for a complete evaluation and assistance if you observe noticeable changes in your urine or if you have health concerns.

CHAPTER ONE

Systems of the Urinary Anatomy and Physiology

Some explanations for why urine may appear hazy can be found by studying the anatomy and physiology of the urinary system. Urine production, storage, and elimination are handled by the urinary system, which is made up of various essential parts.

Kidney systems:

Urine production primarily depends on the kidneys. Urine is produced as a result of them filtering water, extra ions, and waste materials from blood.

Entertainers:

Urine is moved from the kidneys to the bladder by tubes called ureters. Urine travels via the ureters with the assistance of peristalsis contractions.

Bladder

Urine is stored in the muscle bladder until the time comes to release it. Smooth muscle layers in the bladder's lining contract to make urinating easier.

Aurethra:

Urine travels from the bladder to the outside world through a tube called the urethra. The passageway for semen in males during ejaculation is the urethra.

A few of the elements that affect urine's clarity and how it forms are as follows:

The kidneys are where filtration takes place after blood enters through the renal arteries. Retinal tubules receive filtered substances, including water, electrolytes, and waste materials.

Re-entry:

Vital components like water and electrolytes are reabsorbed back into the bloodstream when the filtrate passes through the renal tubules in order to keep the body balanced.

Keep it secret:

The renal tubules actively secrete a number of chemicals, such as medications and waste materials.

urine concentration:

Water is reabsorption in the renal tubules affects urine concentration. It could look hazy if you're dehydrated or have concentrated urine.

Mucous and Cells:

Mucus-producing mucous membranes line the urinary tract. Furthermore, a tiny number of cells may be present in normal pee. Cloudiness, however, can also result from an overabundance of mucus or aberrant cell growth.

White blood cells and other detritus can cause cloudiness when there are bacterial infections in the urinary tract, which includes the bladder and kidneys.

Cloudiness in urine can be caused by crystals and sediments that accumulate in the urine as a result of illnesses such kidney stones and dehydration.

Mucus production and cloudiness may be exacerbated by inflammation of the kidneys, bladder, or urinary tract.

Healthcare providers can identify probable causes of murky urine and devise effective diagnostic and treatment plans by having a thorough understanding of the complex functions of the urinary system. Getting medical counsel is crucial for a complete assessment if someone notices consistent or worrisome changes in the clarity of their pee.

Common Reasons for Perturbative Pee

A number of things can cause cloudy urine; some are very benign, but others might be a sign of a more serious medical condition. Common reasons of murky urine include the following:

Hypohydration:

Dehydration can concentrate urine, which might look hazy. A greater concentration of waste materials and minerals in the urine is caused by inadequate fluid consumption.

A urinary tract infection (UTI) is:

Urinary cloudiness can result from bacterial diseases of the urinary tract, such as cystitis or pyelonephritis. Pain when urinating and frequent urination are common symptoms of urinary tract infections.

Rough Stones:

A contributing factor to cloudy urine is the presence of crystals or particles in the urine, as observed in kidney stones. It can hurt and be uncomfortable to have kidney stones.

STIs, or infections spread through sexual contact:

Urine may seem hazy as a result of certain STDs, including chlamydia and gonorrhea. Itching, drainage, or soreness are possible additional symptoms.

The proteinuric state

The condition known as proteinuria, or too much protein in the urine, can cause cloudiness and be linked to renal issues.

Cystitis, or Bladder Infection

Urine that has cloudiness can be a sign of bladder infections. Urgency, pain, and changes in the color of the urine are among symptoms.

Vaginal Drainage:

Cloudiness in urine can occasionally result from the mixing of vaginal discharge in women. Urine appearance may be impacted by this, but it has nothing to do with the urinary system.

Initial Fluid:

Urine may temporarily become cloudy during sexual activity if seminal fluid that has remained in the urethra mixes with it. Usually, this is nothing to be alarmed about.

Certain Drugs:

Urine clarity and color variations can be brought on by some drugs or supplements. Should you suspect medication-related cloudiness, speak with a healthcare provider.

Urine can seem cloudy or differently during pregnancy due to hormonal changes.

proteinuria orthostatic:

a condition where urine contains protein only while the person is standing up. It is more common in young adults and usually goes away when they lie down.

Chemical Pollutants

Urine that appears murky may be a result of environmental pollutants or chemical exposure.

It is noteworthy to mention that certain meals, like asparagus, can also momentarily alter the color and clarity of urine.

A trip to the doctor is necessary if there are persistent cloudiness or other symptoms, even though occasional cloudiness in the urine may be normal. The underlying cause may be found by doing diagnostic testing, such as urinalysis. It's essential to consult a doctor for a complete evaluation and assistance if you observe noticeable changes in your urine or if you have health concerns.

Signs and Measurements of Particles, sediments, or other materials that impair urine's clarity can be seen visually in cloudy urine. Although hazy urine is a symptom in and of itself, it may also be connected to other indications and symptoms that offer more information about the underlying origin. Cloudy urine can present with the following symptoms and signs:

Rather than seeming clear, the pee is murky, milky, or turbid. A faint haziness to a more noticeable opacity can be found in different degrees of cloudiness.

Modifications in Hue:

Variations in hue may also be present with cloudy urine. Depending on what is causing it, the urine can seem yellow, brown, pink, or green.

Urine may smell different, and if it's murky, the difference in smell might be more apparent. There are various conditions that can be linked to strong or unpleasant smells.

Aches or unease:

Along with murky urine, dysuria pain or discomfort experienced during urination may also exist. With illnesses like urinary tract infections (UTIs), this is typical.

Frequently Needing to Urinate

When urinary tract disorders like bladder infections occur, there may be an increase in the frequency of urinating.

Relevance:

Bladder infections and other related disorders can cause an overwhelming need to urinate even when the bladder is not full.

Sensation that Burns:

Common symptoms of urinary tract infections include burning or stinging while urinating, which may also be accompanied by hazy urine.

Temperature spike:

Urinary tract infections, for example, might cause murky urine to be accompanied by fever. An indication of the body's immunological reaction is an elevated temperature.

Pain in the lower abdomen:

Conditions affecting the bladder or lower urinary system are frequently linked to lower abdominal pain or discomfort.

Back Soreness:

Urea clouding and back pain are two other symptoms of kidney-related disorders, such as kidney stones and infections.

Childhood Urinary Urgency:

Cloudy urine in children may be a sign of a urinary tract infection, especially when combined with increased urgency or frequency of urinating.

Hematuria, or the appearance of blood in urine, Hematuria may be indicated in certain situations by murky urine and visible blood. Urine that has blood in it may turn pink, red, or brown.

Foamy Dilution:

Particularly in cases of proteinuria excessive protein in the urine foamy or frothy urine may be noticed.

It is vital to understand that medical professionals can limit down the possible reasons of hazy urine by looking for a certain combination of symptoms. In order to have a complete evaluation and the right treatment, it is imperative that someone with persistent or worrisome symptoms seek medical attention.

CHAPTER TWO

Identification and Assessment

A methodical approach to determining the underlying reason is necessary for the diagnosis and assessment of hazy urine. The cause of murky urine may be ascertained by medical professionals using a combination of laboratory testing, physical examination, and medical history. In order to diagnose and assess cloudy urine, follow these standard procedures:

Background information on health:

The medical professional will ask about the patient's past health, including any recent diseases, prescription drugs, eating routine, sexual activity, and symptoms related to the urinary system.

Evaluation of the body:

An assessment of general health and the detection of infection, inflammation, or other disorders may be achieved by a physical examination. Abdominal and vaginal exams may be part of the examination.

An analysis of urine

The examination of a urine sample is a vital diagnostic procedure known as urinalysis. Information concerning the existence of substances that might cause cloudiness, such as crystals, white blood cells, blood, and bacteria, can be obtained from it.

Culture of urine:

Urine cultures may be carried out to pinpoint the precise bacteria causing a urinary tract infection (UTI) if one is suspected of having one. Finding the best antibiotic for therapy depends on this.

Research on Imaging:

Magnetic resonance imaging (MRI), computed tomography (CT) scans, ultrasounds, and other imaging procedures may be ordered to visualize the urinary tract in cases with recurrent kidney stones or suspected anatomical abnormalities.

Tests on Blood:

To evaluate renal function, look for indications of infection or inflammation, and find any underlying systemic problems, blood tests may be performed.

An instrument called a cystoscopy, which allows one to see within the bladder and urethra, is a thin, flexible tube with a camera that is placed via the urethra. Direct urinary tract examination may be necessary in specific circumstances.

Examination of the Pelvic Floor:

To evaluate the state of the reproductive organs and locate any possible sources of vaginal discharge that might have an impact on the purity of the urine, a pelvic examination may be performed on females.

A pregnancy test could be carried out if cloudiness in the urine is connected to other symptoms that point to pregnancy.

Consulting with Experts:

Consultation with experts in infectious diseases, gynecology, urology, or nephrology may be advised for additional assessment and treatment, contingent on the results.

The particular diagnostic strategy will be determined by the presumed reason for the murky urine. Sometimes, in order to guarantee a thorough assessment, several examinations and consultations are needed. It is imperative that you get medical help right once, particularly if you have any concomitant symptoms like discomfort, fever, or consistently murky urine. By doing so, the underlying disease can be successfully identified and treated.

The underlying reason of murky urine must be determined by diagnostic testing before treatment may begin. Medical practitioners might suggest suitable treatment strategies after the reason has been identified. Based on the underlying causes, the following are typical treatment approaches for murky urine:

Acute urinary tract infections (UTIs):

Antibiotics: Antibiotics are usually recommended to target specific bacteria if murky urine is the result of a bacterial illness. It's crucial to take antibiotics as directed for the entire recommended course.

Rough Stones:

Pain Relief: Pain from kidney stones can be managed with over-the-counter or prescription pain relief.

An increase in fluid intake can aid in the passage of smaller stones and renal flushing, as drinking lots of water does.

Medication to Assist in Stone Passage: Kidney stone passage may occasionally be aided by prescription drugs that relax the ureter's muscles.

STIs, or infections spread through sexual contact:

Antibiotics are used in the treatment of sexually transmitted infections (STIs), including chlamydia and gonorrhea. It's possible that both partners require treatment.

The proteinuric state

Managing the Primary Condition is Crucial if Proteinuria Is Associated with an Underlying Kidney Disease. Medication and lifestyle adjustments can be necessary for this.

Hypohydration:

Hydration: Consuming more fluids might help reduce cloudiness brought on by dehydration by diluting the urine.

Vaginal Fluid or Seminal Fluid Outflow:

Keeping oneself clean: You can avoid vaginal discharge from clouding your urine by practicing good hygiene.

Men who have had intercourse may find that urinating afterwards helps help remove any seminal fluid that may have remained in the urethra.

proteinuria orthostatic:

Orthostatic proteinuria, which is frequent in young adults, may not require special therapy. Monitoring and lifestyle measures are also important. It might be advised to follow certain lifestyle guidelines, such drinking enough of water and avoiding extended standing.

Control of Supplementary Circumstances:

Particular Therapies: The methods of treatment may change according to the underlying diseases found in diagnostic assessments. This can entail treating inflammatory diseases, controlling illnesses like diabetes, or offering suitable treatments for anatomical difficulties.

Patients experiencing murky urine should make sure they follow their doctor's instructions and finish the recommended course of medication. It is essential to follow up with the healthcare provider if symptoms worsen or persist, or if there are new concerns.

It is not advised to self-diagnose or self-treat, as usual. A precise diagnosis and suitable care catered to the patient's unique medical requirements are ensured while seeking competent medical advice.

Self-care and At-Home Treatments

Although medical intervention is generally necessary to address the underlying cause of cloudy urine, there are certain self-care techniques and home remedies that can help manage symptoms and promote urinary health in general. It's crucial to remember that these actions do not replace expert medical guidance, and anyone who is suffering severe or chronic symptoms should speak with a doctor. Cloudy urine can be treated at home with these natural therapies and self-care advice:

Sustain Your Hydration:

Sustaining urinary health requires drinking enough water. Water consumption lowers urine's viscosity and facilitates the urinary system's cleansing.

The juice of cranberries:

Because it inhibits the adherence of germs to the urinary system, cranberry juice may help prevent UTIs. If you want to stay away from additional sugars, you must use pure, unsweetened cranberry juice.

Refrain from Irritants:

Steer clear of meals, alcohol, caffeine, and spicy beverages that can irritate the urinary system.

Hot Compress:

In order to ease the discomfort brought on by some urinary disorders, like bladder infections, apply a warm compress to the lower abdomen.

Adequate Personal Hygiene:

Reduce your risk of infection by maintaining proper personal cleanliness, especially in the genital area.

Following a Sexual Activity, Urinate:

Urinating after sexual activity is beneficial for both men and women in terms of removing any bacteria that may have entered the urinary system.

Maintain an Appropriate Nutrition:

Overall health, especially urinary health, is supported by eating a balanced diet high in fruits, vegetables, and whole grains.

Steer clear of holding urine:

Urinary stasis and infection risk can be minimized by routinely emptying the bladder and avoiding extended durations of retaining urine.

Exercises for the pelvic floor:

Strengthening the muscles supporting urine function can be achieved through pelvic floor exercises, such Kegel exercises.

Lessen Tension:

Persistent stress has an effect on the urinary system as well as general health. Utilizing stress-reduction methods like meditation or deep breathing could be helpful.

Use of irritant products should be limited.

The urinary system might get irritated by using perfumed feminine hygiene products, bubble baths, and harsh soaps.

Maintain a Healthful BMI:

Urinary problems may arise as a result of obesity. Urinary health may be supported by maintaining a healthy weight through balanced eating and frequent exercise.

It is important to keep in mind that these self-care techniques are helpful and could be beneficial in specific circumstances. Seeking professional medical assistance is necessary for a comprehensive evaluation and proper treatment, though, if murky urine continues or is accompanied by other worrisome symptoms. When medical attention is necessary, home remedies shouldn't be used in place of or in addition to it.

Adaptation Techniques and Psychological Health

Changes in the way you pee, such foggy pee, can be alarming and have an effect on your mental health. When it comes to handling the emotional side of urinary difficulties, coping mechanisms can be quite important. For emotional health, consider the following coping mechanisms and advice:

Obtain Expert Advice:

Get the help you need by speaking with a medical expert to identify the reason behind hazy urine. Anxiety can be reduced by knowing what the underlying cause is.

Get Knowledgeable:

Get information on hazy urine's causes and remedies. Information helps people feel more empowered and less uncertain.

CHAPTER THREE

Transparent Communication

Talk about your worries and emotions with your partner, a close friend, or your healthcare provider. Being open with one another can ease feelings of loneliness and offer emotional support.

Employ Stress Reduction Techniques:

Apply stress-reduction strategies to your everyday life, such as mindfulness, meditation, or deep breathing. Total well-being is influenced by stress management.

Join Conversational Support Groups:

Establish a connection with people who could be going through comparable health difficulties. Online discussion boards and support groups offer a space for exchanging stories and getting support.

Put on Some Exercise:

Mood and emotional well-being can be enhanced by regular exercise. Select pursuits that suit your level of fitness and that you enjoy.

Sustain a Healthy Way of Living:

To enhance general well-being, one should have a healthy lifestyle that includes frequent exercise, a balanced diet, and enough sleep.

Set sensible objectives:

To manage your health, set attainable objectives. Condense more ambitious objectives into manageable steps.

Put Self-Care First:

Set aside time for enjoyable and calming self-care activities. For emotional health, self-care is crucial, whether it takes the form of reading, taking a bath, or going outside.

Remain informed:

Be knowledgeable about your medical condition and your course of therapy. A person's ability to actively engage in their care is enhanced by knowledge.

Continue to See the Bright Side:

Praise the good things in life and give thanks for them to cultivate an optimistic outlook. Exercise appreciation to help you turn your attention to the good things in life.

Construct a Support Network:

Keep a network of friends, family, and medical professionals who are all supportive of you. The impact on mental well-being of having a solid support system can be substantial.

Examine professional counseling:

See a mental health professional for support if necessary. When faced with difficult circumstances, counseling can offer coping mechanisms and emotional support.

It is crucial to note that coping tactics differ across individuals and that you should seek out approaches that align with your personal requirements and preferences. A comprehensive approach to well-being incorporates both seeking professional advice and preserving open communication. Do not be reluctant to contact mental health specialists who are trained in helping people with health issues if emotional anguish continues.

Signs to Look Out for and When to Get Help

Some red flags point to the need for immediate medical attention, even though cloudy urine is occasionally harmless and transient. Seeking medical attention right away is crucial if you have any of the following signs or situations in addition to cloudy urine:

Very Bad Pain:

A urinary tract obstruction or kidney stones are two more serious underlying conditions that may be indicated by intense pain, especially in the lower abdomen, pelvis, or back.

Temperature spike:

If accompanied by cloudy urine, a fever may indicate an infection, and treatment for a urinary tract infection (UTI) or other systemic infection is necessary right away.

Blood in the Pee (Hematuria):

It may indicate a more serious problem like kidney stones, infection, or damage to the kidneys or bladder if your urine is not only hazy but also shows signs of visible blood.

Sustaining Cloud Cover:

If your urine still appears cloudy after trying home cures or altering your water intake, there may be a more serious problem that needs to be checked out by a doctor.

A higher amplitude and intensity:

Urine that is cloudy and that you need to urinate more frequently or urgently could be signs of a urinary tract infection or other urinary problems.

Shade Shifts in Urine:

It may be an indication of the presence of blood or other dangerous materials if your urine is not only hazy but also dark (brown or reddish-brown).

Significant Pain When Urinating:

An infection of the urinary tract or other problems affecting the urinary system may be indicated by pain, burning, or discomfort during urinating, especially if it goes on.

Background of Renal Disorders:

Cloudy urine may indicate an aggravation or complication that needs to be addressed if you have a history of renal disease or are at risk for developing kidney problems.

Correlated Illnesses in Particular Groups:

If you have murky urine along with other symptoms, you should get medical assistance right once if you belong to a specific group, such as elderly people or pregnant women.

Any recent catheterizations or surgeries

Urine that appears hazy may be an indication of possible problems if you have recently had surgery, required urinary catheterization, or suffered any urinary tract trauma.

You must get medical assistance right away if you experience any of these warning signs or have concerns about your health. Depending on the underlying reason of murky urine and related symptoms, a medical professional can perform a comprehensive evaluation, order relevant tests, and administer the proper treatment. Delaying getting help or ignoring warning signs could exacerbate the underlying issue or cause further problems.

Doubtful Pee in Certain Groups

Multitudes of people can experience cloudy urine, thus different groups may need to take different precautions. Cloudy urine may have different consequences for the following specific populations:

Those that are pregnant:

Changes in hormones, increased vaginal discharge, or urinary tract infections (UTIs) can all contribute to cloudy urine in pregnant women. It is important for expectant mothers to speak with their healthcare professional and treat any changes in their urine as soon as possible.

Youngs:

Dehydration or a urinary tract infection (UTI) could be indicated by cloudy urine in children. Parents should be alert to changes in their child's urine patterns and seek medical assistance if necessary, as children may not always be able to appropriately explain their concerns.

Older People:

Seniors who have cloudy urine may be suffering from dehydration, urinary tract infections, or adverse drug reactions. Urinary symptoms in the elderly should be rapidly evaluated due to immune system changes associated with aging.

People whose immune systems are compromised:

urinary tract infections and other urinary problems may be more common in people whose immune systems are weakened, such as those receiving chemotherapy or dealing with diseases like HIV/AIDS. This group should get treatment for cloudy urine right away.

Diabetes sufferers:

Urinary tract infections are made more likely by diabetes, and this can lead to hazy pee. Diabetes can also cause kidney-related complications that can alter a person's urine habits.

Post-Optional Individuals:

Postoperative medication, fluid balance changes, and catheter use are some of the factors that may contribute to cloudy urine following surgery. Urinary changes must be reported to the healthcare team by postoperative patients.

Those who suffer from renal diseases:

Urine clarity can alter for those who already have kidney disease, such as chronic kidney disease. For this group, cloudy urine should be assessed by a medical practitioner as it could indicate a worsening of the kidney disease.

People Who've Had Urinary Stones in the Past:

Renal stone patients may have frequent episodes of cloudy urine, particularly during stone formation or passage episodes. To stop a stone from coming back, it could be advised to drink enough water and make dietary changes.

Cloudy urine that is accompanied by warning signs or worrisome symptoms requires immediate medical attention in all special populations. In order to address the unique needs and concerns of each population, healthcare providers can tailor treatment plans, order necessary tests, and conduct appropriate assessments. Optimal urinary health in these specific populations is facilitated by proactive management and routine follow-ups.

Let's sum up by saying that there are a number of reasons why urine can appear cloudy, from mild, transient ailments to more serious underlying medical conditions. Urine clouding frequently indicates the presence of particles, sediments, or other substances that are changing the urine's composition.

A number of medical conditions, including kidney stones, dehydration, STIs, urinary tract infections (UTIs), and others, can cause cloudy urine. A person's diet, medications, and way of life can all have an impact.

It's crucial to be aware of any related symptoms, like pain, fever, or altered urination patterns, when dealing with cloudy urine. Symptoms that should alert people to seek medical attention right away include severe pain, blood in the urine, or persistent cloudiness.

Urinalysis, physical examination, medical history, and, if required, further tests like imaging studies or cultures are all part of the comprehensive process for diagnosing and treating cloudy urine.

How to treat cloudy urine depends on what's causing it. Infection treatment with antibiotics, kidney stone pain relief, lifestyle changes, or treating particular medical conditions could all be part of this.

Urinary health can be promoted by using natural remedies and self-care practices like drinking plenty of water, practicing good hygiene, and leading a healthy lifestyle. The key to managing the emotional impact of urinary changes is emotional well-being and coping strategies.

Specialized approaches to diagnosis and management are crucial in special populations, such as the elderly, children, pregnant women, and people with certain medical conditions. Considerations may differ depending on the case.

To summarize, if murky urine is present along with worrisome symptoms, it is important to take it seriously. For best urinary health and general well-being, seek medical attention as soon as possible, comprehend the underlying causes, and adhere to prescribed treatments. Comprehensive care and suitable management of cloudy urine are ensured by regular communication with healthcare professionals.

THE END